Isometric exercise

A Guide on the Use of Isometric Exercises Effectively for Building Muscle and Limiting Muscle Loss

Thulani Nkosi

Table of Contents

CHAPTER ONE
Introduction to Isometric Exercise

Isometric exercise, a lesser-known yet highly effective form of strength training, revolves around the concept of muscle contraction without visible movement. Unlike traditional exercises that involve dynamic motions such as lifting or bending, isometric exercises entail holding a static position, challenging your muscles to generate force without altering their length.

The term "isometric" is derived from the Greek words "isos," meaning equal, and "metron," meaning measure. In essence, during isometric exercises, the muscles remain at a constant length, as they work against an immovable force or object. This unique approach to resistance training offers a myriad of benefits, making it a valuable addition to fitness routines for individuals of various ages and fitness levels.

Isometric exercises involve contracting muscles without changing the joint angle or experiencing visible movement.

This static nature distinguishes them from dynamic exercises.

By isolating specific muscle groups and holding positions, isometric exercises effectively engage and strengthen targeted areas. This can be particularly advantageous for enhancing stability and promoting balanced muscle development.

One of the standout features of isometric exercises is their accessibility. They can be performed virtually anywhere, requiring minimal to no equipment. This versatility makes them an attractive option for those seeking a practical and time-efficient workout.

Isometric exercises offer a time-efficient workout solution. Even brief sessions can yield significant benefits, making them suitable for individuals with busy schedules.

Isometric exercises are generally considered safe, especially for individuals with joint concerns or those recovering from injuries. Their adaptability allows for customization based on individual fitness levels, ensuring a low-impact yet effective workout.

Whether you're a fitness enthusiast looking to diversify your routine or someone exploring gentle yet impactful strength training, isometric exercises might just be the key to unlocking a new dimension of physical fitness.

Benefits of Isometric Exercise

Isometric exercises target specific muscle groups and promote strength development. They help build muscular endurance, allowing muscles to sustain contractions for longer periods.

Isometric exercises can be time-efficient, as they often require shorter durations compared to dynamic exercises. Quick sessions can provide significant benefits, making them suitable for individuals with busy schedules.

Isometric exercises are generally low-impact and put less stress on the joints compared to some dynamic exercises. They can be a safer option for individuals with joint issues or those recovering from injuries.

Holding static positions requires concentration, fostering a mind-body connection during workouts. The focus required in isometric exercises can contribute to improved mental clarity and stress reduction.

Isometric exercises are often incorporated into rehabilitation programs for their gentle yet effective nature. They can aid in preventing injuries by strengthening muscles and improving joint stability.

Isometric exercises mimic real-world activities, promoting functional fitness by improving the body's ability to perform daily tasks.

CHAPTER TWO
Isometric Contractions

Isometric contractions are a type of muscle contraction where the muscle generates tension and exerts force without undergoing a visible change in length. In simpler terms, during an isometric contraction, the muscle remains static, and there is no movement at the joint.

Characteristics of isometric contractions include:

Static Position:

Isometric contractions involve holding a position or maintaining a specific joint angle without any visible movement. The muscle contracts, but the length of the muscle does not change during the contraction.

No Joint Movement:

Unlike dynamic exercises where muscles lengthen (eccentric) or shorten (concentric), isometric contractions do not involve joint movement. The muscle contracts against an immovable force or object.

Muscle Engagement:

Isometric contractions engage specific muscle groups without the need for dynamic movements. Muscles generate tension and force during the contraction, leading to increased activation of motor units.

Strength Building:

Isometric contractions are effective for building strength, particularly in specific muscle groups. The sustained tension during isometric exercises contributes to muscle endurance and strength development.

Applications in Exercise:

Isometric contractions are commonly used in exercises such as planks, wall sits, and static holds. They can be integrated into strength training routines to target and isolate particular muscles.

Joint Safety:

Isometric contractions are generally considered low-impact and put less stress on the joints compared to some dynamic exercises. This makes them suitable for individuals with joint concerns or those recovering from injuries.

Rehabilitation: Isometric contractions are often incorporated into rehabilitation programs due to their controlled nature. They can be used to gently strengthen muscles without subjecting joints to excessive movement.

Increased Muscle Coordination: Isometric contractions contribute to improved muscle coordination and recruitment of motor units within the muscle. This can enhance overall muscle function and performance.

Versatility:

Isometric contractions can be adapted to various fitness levels and goals. They are versatile and can be included in different workout routines for targeted muscle engagement.

Examples of Isometric Contractions:

Holding a squat position without moving up or down.

Keeping the arms at a specific angle without bending or straightening.

Maintaining a specific yoga pose without transitioning to another position.

Types of Muscle Contractions

Muscle contractions can be categorized into three main types based on the changes in muscle length and the resulting movement at the joints. These types are:

Concentric Contractions:

During a concentric contraction, the muscle shortens as it generates force against resistance. In a bicep curl, the concentric phase occurs when you lift the weight toward your shoulder, and the biceps muscle shortens.

Eccentric Contractions:

Eccentric contractions involve the lengthening of a muscle as it generates force against resistance. It's often the controlled lowering phase of a movement. Using the same bicep curl example, the eccentric phase occurs when you lower the weight back down, and the biceps muscle lengthens.

Isometric Contractions:

Isometric contractions occur when the muscle generates force without changing in length, resulting in no visible movement at the joint. Holding a plank position or pushing against an immovable object, where the muscles are contracted, but there is no joint movement.

Dynamic exercise

Dynamic exercise refers to physical activities that involve a range of motion and repetitive muscle contractions, leading to visible joint movement. These exercises typically include both concentric (muscle shortening) and eccentric (muscle lengthening) contractions, creating dynamic movements. Dynamic exercises are often associated with activities that require flexibility, strength, and endurance. Characteristics and examples of dynamic exercises:

Characteristics of Dynamic Exercise:

Dynamic exercises involve the movement of joints through a full range of motion.

Both concentric and eccentric muscle contractions occur during dynamic exercises.

Dynamic exercises often involve repetitive actions, such as multiple repetitions of a specific movement or exercise.

These exercises typically engage multiple muscle groups and joints simultaneously.

Many dynamic exercises have a cardiovascular component, increasing heart rate and respiratory activity.

Dynamic exercises often mimic real-world movements, promoting functional fitness and overall athleticism.

Examples of Dynamic Exercises:

Squats:

Squats involve bending the knees and hips to lower the body and then returning to the starting position. This exercise engages the muscles of the lower body, including the quadriceps, hamstrings, and glutes.

Running:

Running is a dynamic cardiovascular exercise that involves repetitive movements of the legs and engages various muscle groups, including the quadriceps, hamstrings, calves, and hip flexors.

Push-Ups:

Push-ups require the arms to move through a full range of motion, engaging the chest, shoulders, triceps, and core muscles.

Jumping Jacks:

Jumping jacks involve simultaneous jumping and arm movements, engaging the legs, core, and shoulders.

Lunges:

Lunges involve stepping forward or backward and bending the knees, engaging the quadriceps, hamstrings, and glutes.

Cycling:

Cycling is a dynamic exercise that involves repetitive pedaling motions, engaging the muscles of the legs and providing cardiovascular benefits.

Burpees:

Burpees combine several movements, including a squat, push-up, and jump, providing a full-body dynamic exercise.

Swimming:

Swimming involves dynamic movements of the arms and legs, engaging various muscle groups while providing a low-impact cardiovascular workout.

CHAPTER THREE
How Isometric Differs from Dynamic Exercises

Isometric exercises and dynamic exercises represent two distinct approaches to strength training, and they differ primarily in the way muscles contract and the resulting joint movement.

How isometric exercises differ from dynamic exercises:

Muscle Contraction:

Isometric Exercises: Muscles contract without visible movement at the joint.

The length of the muscle remains constant during the contraction.

Dynamic Exercises: Muscles undergo either concentric (shortening) or eccentric (lengthening) contractions, resulting in visible movement at the joint.

Joint Movement:

Isometric Exercises: There is no joint movement during isometric contractions. The joint angle remains constant as the muscles generate force.

Dynamic Exercises: Joint movement occurs as muscles contract and move bones. This movement can be in various planes, such as flexion, extension, abduction, or adduction, depending on the exercise.

Examples:

Isometric Exercises: Holding a plank, wall sit, or static yoga poses where the position is maintained without joint movement.

Dynamic Exercises: Bicep curls, squats, push-ups, and other exercises involving visible joint movement as muscles contract and relax.

Strength and Endurance:

Isometric Exercises: Effective for building static strength and endurance. Muscles work against resistance without changing length.

Dynamic Exercises: Promote strength throughout a range of motion and can also enhance muscular endurance, depending on the number of repetitions and sets.

Specificity:

Isometric Exercises: Often target specific muscle groups without the need for joint movement. Ideal for isolating and strengthening particular muscles.

Dynamic Exercises: Engage multiple muscle groups and joints, promoting overall functional fitness and movement patterns.

Equipment and Setup:

Isometric Exercises: Typically require little to no equipment. Exercises can be performed using body weight or minimal props.

Dynamic Exercises: May involve various types of equipment, such as dumbbells, resistance bands, or machines, depending on the exercise.

Adaptability:

Isometric Exercises: Can be adapted for individuals with joint concerns or limited mobility since there is no dynamic movement.

Dynamic Exercises: Provide a broad range of movement and can be adapted for different fitness levels and goals.

Time Under Tension:

Isometric Exercises: Tension is sustained throughout the duration of the contraction, providing a constant challenge to the muscles.

Dynamic Exercises: Time under tension varies as muscles contract and relax during different phases of the exercise.

Muscles Involved in Isometric Exercises

Isometric exercises can engage a variety of muscle groups, and the specific muscles involved depend on the nature of the isometric exercise.

Core Muscles:

The core muscles make up a group of muscles in the torso that provide stability and support for the spine, pelvis, and overall body. A strong core is essential for maintaining good posture, preventing injuries, and facilitating various physical activities. The core muscles include:

Rectus Abdominis: It is located at the frontal abdominal muscles. It is responsible for flexing the spine, commonly known as the "six-pack" muscles. Exercises include: crunches, sit-ups, leg raises.

Obliques: It is located at the side muscles on either side of the torso. It Involved in trunk rotation, lateral flexion, and providing stability. Exercise include russian twists, side planks, oblique crunches.

Transverse Abdominis (TVA): It is located at the deep abdominal muscles that wrap around the torso. It provides core stability and helps compress the abdominal contents. Exercise include planks, vacuum exercises (pulling the belly button toward the spine), pelvic tilts.

Erector Spinae: It is located at the muscles along the spine in the lower back. It is responsible for extending the spine and providing support. Exercise include lack extensions, good mornings, deadlifts.

Multifidus: It is located at the deep muscles along the spine. it stabilizes the spine and helps control movement. Exercises include bird dogs, cat-cow stretches.

Pelvic Floor Muscles: It is located at the muscles at the base of the pelvis. It supports the pelvic organs, contributes to urinary and bowel control. Exercise include kegel exercises.

Quadriceps:

the quadriceps are a group of four muscles located at the front of the thigh. They play a key role in lower body movement, helping to extend the knee and flex the hip. The quadriceps muscles are essential for activities such as walking, running, jumping, and standing up from a seated position. They include the rectus femoris, vastus lateralis, vastus medialis, and vastus intermedius. Exercises like squats, leg presses, lunges, leg extensions, and step-ups target the quadriceps and help strengthen and tone the muscles for improved functionality and performance in various activities.

Gluteal Muscles:

The gluteal muscles, commonly known as the glutes, are a group of muscles located in the buttocks. The main muscles in this group are the gluteus maximus, gluteus medius, and gluteus minimus. They play a crucial role in various movements of the hip and thigh, contributing to overall lower body strength, stability, and functional mobility. The gluteus maximus is the largest and outermost muscle, responsible for hip extension and thigh abduction. The gluteus medius and minimus, situated on the outer surface of the pelvis, contribute to hip abduction, stabilization, and internal rotation.

Exercises such as squats, deadlifts, hip thrusts, lunges, and specific isolation exercises target the gluteal muscles. Strengthening these muscles is important for activities like standing, walking, running, and maintaining pelvic stability. A well-developed and functional gluteal region is not only aesthetically pleasing but also crucial for overall lower body strength and injury prevention.

Hamstrings:

The hamstrings are a group of muscles located on the back of the thigh, consisting of the biceps femoris, semimembranosus, and semitendinosus. These muscles play a vital role in various lower body movements, including knee flexion and hip extension. Functions of the hamstrings include bending the knee, extending the hip, decelerating leg swing during walking or running, and stabilizing the knee joint.

Exercises that target the hamstrings include dead lifts, leg curls, good mornings, Romanian deadlifts, and lunges. Strengthening the hamstrings is crucial for balanced lower body strength, injury prevention, and overall athletic performance. Incorporating a variety of exercises helps ensure comprehensive development and functional flexibility in the hamstring muscles.

Deltoids and Shoulder Muscles:

The deltoids and shoulder muscles are crucial for upper body movement and stability. The deltoids have three parts: anterior, medial, and posterior, responsible for lifting the arms forward, sideways, and backward, respectively. Additionally, the rotator cuff and trapezius contribute to shoulder function. Exercises like shoulder press, lateral raises, and rows help strengthen these muscles, promoting overall upper body strength and functionality.

Chest and Triceps:

The chest muscles (pectoralis major) and triceps are key upper body muscles. The chest is responsible for movements like pushing and bringing the arms across the chest. Triceps, located at the back of the arm, are crucial for straightening the elbow. They often work together in exercises like bench press and push-ups. Strengthening these muscle groups enhances overall upper body strength and supports various pushing movements.

Biceps and Forearms:

The biceps, located in the front of the upper arm, help bend the elbow. Forearms, between the wrist and elbow, assist with gripping and wrist movements. Strengthening exercises for biceps include curls, and for forearms, wrist curls. Both muscle groups collaborate for tasks like lifting and gripping objects.

Back Muscles:

Back muscles are located along the spine and contribute to posture, stability, and movement. Key muscles include the latissimus dorsi (lats), trapezius, and rhomboids. Exercises like pull-ups, rows, and deadlifts strengthen the back. A strong back is crucial for daily activities and supports overall upper body strength.

Calf Muscles:

Calf muscles are found in the lower leg, and the main ones are the gastrocnemius and soleus. They help lift the heel and assist in walking and running. Calf raises and walking on tiptoes are common exercises to strengthen the calves. Developing strong calf muscles contributes to lower leg stability and overall mobility.

Neck Muscles:

Neck muscles, including the sternocleidomastoid and trapezius, support head movement. They help with turning, tilting, and nodding the head. Exercises like neck tilts and rotations strengthen and improve flexibility. Strong neck muscles contribute to good posture and overall upper body stability.

CHAPTER FOUR
Major Muscle Groups

The human body is composed of numerous muscles, and they can be broadly categorized into major muscle groups based on their location and function. Working these major muscle groups is essential for overall strength, stability, and functional movement. Major muscle groups in the body:

Chest Muscles (Pectorals):

Functions: Responsible for shoulder movement, arm flexion, and adduction of the arms.

Exercises: Bench press, push-ups, chest fly.

Back Muscles:

Latissimus Dorsi (Lats): Located on the sides of the back, responsible for arm extension and adduction.

Rhomboids: Between the shoulder blades, involved in shoulder blade retraction.

Trapezius: Upper back and neck, responsible for shoulder and neck movement.

Exercises: Pull-ups, rows, deadlifts.

Shoulder Muscles (Deltoids):

Anterior Deltoid: Front part, responsible for shoulder flexion.

Medial Deltoid: Middle part, involved in shoulder abduction.

Posterior Deltoid: Back part, responsible for shoulder extension.

Exercises: Shoulder press, lateral raises, front raises.

Arms:

Biceps Brachii: Located on the front of the upper arm, responsible for elbow flexion.

Triceps Brachii: Located on the back of the upper arm, responsible for elbow extension.

Exercises: Bicep curls, tricep dips, skull crushers.

Abdominals (Core Muscles):

Rectus Abdominis: Frontal abdominal muscles, responsible for flexing the spine.

Obliques: Side muscles, involved in trunk rotation and lateral flexion.

Transverse Abdominis: Deep abdominal muscles, contributing to core stability.

Exercises: Crunches, planks, Russian twists.

Leg Muscles:

Quadriceps: Located on the front of the thigh, responsible for knee extension.

Hamstrings: Located on the back of the thigh, responsible for knee flexion.

Gluteal Muscles (Glutes): Muscles of the buttocks, responsible for hip extension.

Calves (Gastrocnemius and Soleus): Located at the back of the lower leg, responsible for ankle plantar flexion.

Exercises: Squats, lunges, leg press, calf raises.

Hip Muscles:

Hip Flexors: Muscles that allow hip flexion.

Hip Adductors and Abductors: Responsible for moving the legs toward and away from the midline.

Exercises: Hip flexor stretches, leg raises, side leg lifts.

Pelvic Floor Muscles:

Pelvic Floor: Muscles that support the pelvic organs and contribute to urinary and bowel control.

Exercises: Kegel exercises, pelvic tilts.

Isometric Exercises for Beginners

Isometric exercises are a great choice for beginners as they provide a low-impact way to build strength and stability without the need for extensive movement. Isometric exercises involve contracting muscles without changing the length of the muscle or joint angle.

Isometric exercises:

Plank:

Start in a push-up position, or on your forearms, and hold the position with a straight back and engaged core.

Wall Sit:

Stand with your back against a wall and lower your body into a seated position, as if sitting in an invisible chair. Hold the position with your thighs parallel to the ground.

Static Lunges:

Step one foot forward into a lunge position, keeping the back leg straight.

Hold the position, engaging your leg muscles. Switch legs and repeat.

Leg Raise Hold:

Lie on your back and lift your legs a few inches off the ground, keeping them straight. Hold the position, engaging your core.

Isometric Bicep Curl:

Sit or stand with a resistance band or light weights in hand. Curl your arms to a 90-degree angle and hold the position.

Chair Squat Hold:

Stand in front of a chair with your feet shoulder-width apart. Lower your body into a squat position and hold the pose just above the chair without sitting.

Isometric Chest Press:

Sit or stand and press your palms together in front of your chest with resistance. Push your hands together for a few seconds, engaging your chest muscles.

Isometric Shoulder Press:

Sit or stand with your arms bent at 90 degrees. Push your hands upward and hold for a few seconds.

CHAPTER FIVE
Advanced Isometric Exercises

Advanced isometric exercises challenge your muscles and require a higher level of strength and stability. Before attempting advanced isometric exercises, ensure you have a strong foundation in basic exercises and good overall fitness. Advanced isometric exercises:

Planche Progression:

Lift your feet off the ground and lean forward, balancing on your hands.

Progress from tuck planche to full planche.

L-Sit:

Sit on the ground and lift your legs straight out in front of you, forming an "L" shape with your body. Keep your hands on the ground beside your hips.

Human Flag:

Hold onto a vertical pole and lift your body horizontally, keeping it parallel to the ground. Requires significant upper body and core strength.

Front Lever:

Hang from a bar and extend your body horizontally, parallel to the ground, by engaging your back and core muscles.

Horse Stance:

A martial arts-inspired stance where you lower your body into a deep squat and hold the position, engaging your leg muscles.

Plank Variations:

Experiment with challenging plank variations, such as one-arm plank, side plank with leg raise, or elevated plank.

Handstand Hold:

Balance on your hands in a handstand position against a wall or freestanding. Focus on engaging your entire body.

RKC Plank:

In a plank position, squeeze your glutes, engage your core, and create tension throughout your body. This intensifies the standard plank.

Yoga Asanas:

Yoga poses like the crow pose, headstand, or handstand involve isometric holds and advanced balance.

Isometric Pull-Up Holds:

During a pull-up, pause at different points, such as chin over the bar or midway down, and hold the position.

Incorporating isometric exercises

Incorporating isometric exercises into your routine can enhance strength, stability, and overall fitness. How to integrate isometrics effectively:

Warm-Up:

Begin with a dynamic warm-up to increase blood flow and prepare your muscles for exercise. Include light cardio, joint mobility exercises, and dynamic stretches.

Identify Target Areas:

Determine the muscle groups you want to focus on. Isometrics can be applied to various body parts, including the core, upper body, and lower body.

Select Isometric Exercises:

Choose isometric exercises that match your fitness level and goals. For beginners, include foundational exercises like planks, wall sits, or static lunges.

Integrate Isometrics:

Add isometric holds into your existing workout routine. For example, pause at the bottom of a squat, hold a plank position, or incorporate isometric contractions into your strength training exercises.

Progressive Overload:

Gradually increase the duration of your isometric holds or the intensity of the exercises. Progression ensures continued challenge and improvement.

Combine with Dynamic Movements:

Pair isometric exercises with dynamic movements. For instance, follow a plank with push-ups or include isometric holds between sets of traditional strength exercises.

Full-Body Integration:

Incorporate full-body isometric exercises like yoga or Pilates. These practices often involve a combination of static poses and dynamic movements.

Active Recovery:

Use isometric exercises as active recovery during rest days. Gentle isometric stretches or poses can help maintain mobility and promote recovery.

Mind-Muscle Connection:

Focus on the mind-muscle connection during isometric holds. Concentrate on engaging the target muscles and maintaining proper form throughout the hold.

Consistency:

Consistency is crucial for seeing results. Aim to include isometric exercises 2-3 times per week for optimal benefits.

Listen to Your Body:

Pay attention to your body's signals. If you experience pain or discomfort beyond normal muscle fatigue, adjust the intensity or consult with a fitness professional.

Cool Down and Stretch:

Finish your workout with a cool-down and stretching routine to improve flexibility and reduce muscle tension.

Equipment and Tools for Isometric Training

Isometric training often requires minimal equipment, making it accessible for various fitness levels and settings.

Some equipment and tools used for isometric training:

Bodyweight:

Bodyweight exercises are fundamental for isometric training and include movements like planks, wall sits, and static lunges. Easily accessible, requires no additional equipment, and can be done anywhere.

Resistance Bands:

Elastic bands that provide resistance during exercises. Enhances the intensity of isometric exercises, versatile for various muscle groups, and easy to carry.

TRX Suspension Trainer:

Straps with handles that can be anchored to a door frame or sturdy structure for bodyweight exercises. Allows for a wide range of isometric and dynamic exercises, enhances stability, and targets multiple muscle groups.

Yoga Mat:

Cushioned mat for floor exercises and stretches. Provides comfort during isometric holds, especially on hard surfaces, and supports various bodyweight movements.

Stability Ball:

Inflatable ball used for exercises that engage core stability. Adds instability to isometric exercises, particularly for the core, and enhances balance and coordination.

Grip Strengtheners:

Handheld devices designed to improve grip strength. Targets forearm muscles and hand strength, beneficial for isometric exercises involving grip.

Isometric Exercise Device:

Specialized equipment designed for isometric training, providing resistance for muscle engagement without joint movement. Allows for targeted isometric exercises with controlled resistance.

Walls or Poles:

Fixed surfaces used for stability during exercises like wall sits or isometric pushes and pulls. Easily accessible and provides support for various isometric movements.

Kettle bells or Dumbbells:

Weighted equipment used to add resistance to isometric exercises. Increases the challenge for strength-building isometric movements, such as static lunges or holds.

Pull-Up Bar:

Horizontal bar for pull-up exercises. Engages various muscle groups during isometric holds, especially for the upper body.

Timer or Stopwatch:

Devices to measure the duration of isometric holds. Helps track progress and maintain consistency during isometric training.

Plyo Box:

Sturdy box for various exercises, including step-ups and box jumps. Adds height and variety to isometric exercises, especially for lower body strength.

CHAPTER SIX
Mistakes to Avoid

Avoiding common mistakes is crucial to ensuring a safe and effective isometric training routine.

Some mistakes to be aware of and avoid:

Poor Form:

Allowing improper form during isometric exercises. Focus on maintaining correct posture and alignment. Proper form ensures effective muscle engagement and reduces the risk of injury.

Holding Breath:

Holding your breath during isometric holds. Breathe regularly and deeply. Oxygen is essential for muscle function, and proper breathing helps stabilize your core.

Overdoing It:

Holding isometric exercises for too long or using excessive resistance. Start with shorter durations and gradually increase as your strength improves. Use an appropriate level of resistance to prevent strain.

Neglecting Warm-Up:

Skipping a proper warm-up before isometric training. Warm up your muscles with light cardio and dynamic stretches. This helps prevent injuries and prepares your body for the workout.

Ignoring Full-Body Engagement:

Focusing only on specific muscle groups and neglecting full-body engagement. Ensure that your entire body is engaged during isometric exercises. This promotes overall stability and strength.

Lack of Progression:

Sticking to the same level of difficulty without progressing. Gradually increase the duration of holds or resistance to challenge your muscles and promote continuous improvement.

Not Listening to Your Body:

Ignoring pain or discomfort. Pay attention to your body. Discomfort is normal, but sharp pain could indicate an issue. Adjust your form or intensity accordingly.

Inconsistency:

Inconsistently incorporating isometric training into your routine. Make isometric exercises a regular part of your workout routine for consistent progress and benefits.

Relying Solely on Isometrics:

Depending exclusively on isometric exercises for a well-rounded fitness routine. Combine isometrics with dynamic exercises for balanced strength, flexibility, and cardiovascular fitness.

Ignoring Recovery:

Neglecting post-workout recovery. Include stretching, cool-down exercises, and rest days in your routine to facilitate muscle recovery and reduce the risk of overtraining.

Using Incorrect Equipment:

Using inappropriate or unsafe equipment for isometric exercises. Choose equipment that suits your fitness level and the specific requirements of the exercise. Ensure proper setup and stability.

Health Considerations

Before starting any exercise program, including isometric training, it's essential to consider your health and any potential limitations. Health considerations to keep in mind:

Existing Medical Conditions:

If you have any pre-existing medical conditions, such as heart problems, joint issues, or musculoskeletal conditions, consult with your healthcare provider before beginning isometric training.

Injuries:

If you have any recent injuries or chronic pain, especially in the joints or muscles, it's crucial to seek advice from a healthcare professional. Isometric exercises can impact certain areas, and modifications may be necessary.

Blood Pressure:

Isometric exercises can temporarily increase blood pressure. If you have high blood pressure or cardiovascular issues, consult your doctor before engaging in isometric training, and monitor your blood pressure regularly during workouts.

Pregnancy:

Pregnant individuals should consult with their healthcare provider before starting or continuing any exercise routine.

Isometric exercises that involve lying on the back may not be suitable in later stages of pregnancy.

Age:

As we age, joint health and flexibility may vary. Ensure that isometric exercises are appropriate for your age and fitness level. Older adults may need to modify certain exercises to accommodate their capabilities.

Orthopedic Considerations:

Individuals with orthopedic conditions, such as arthritis or osteoporosis, should be cautious with certain isometric exercises. Seek guidance from a healthcare professional or physical therapist.

Medications:

Some medications may affect exercise performance or response. Inform your healthcare provider of any medications you are taking to ensure there are no contraindications with isometric training.

Fitness Level:

Tailor your isometric training to your current fitness level. Beginners should start with simpler exercises and gradually progress. Avoid pushing yourself too hard, especially if you are just starting or returning to exercise.

Hydration and Nutrition:

Adequate hydration and nutrition are important for overall health and exercise performance. Ensure you are well-hydrated before and during your workout, and consider your nutritional needs based on your activity level.

Rest and Recovery:

Allow sufficient time for rest and recovery between workouts. Overtraining can lead to fatigue, increased injury risk, and decreased performance.

Consultation with Professionals:

If you are uncertain about your health or how isometric training may impact you, consider consulting with fitness professionals, such as personal trainers or physical therapists, who can provide guidance based on your individual needs.

CHAPTER SEVEN
Conclusion

Isometric training offers a valuable and accessible approach to building strength, stability, and overall fitness. Whether you're a beginner or an advanced fitness enthusiast, incorporating isometric exercises into your routine can bring numerous benefits.

Isometric exercises can be done virtually anywhere, requiring minimal or no equipment. This versatility makes them suitable for individuals with various fitness levels and preferences.

Isometric training effectively targets specific muscle groups, promoting strength and endurance. It complements dynamic exercises and can contribute to a well-rounded strength training routine.

Isometric exercises are generally low-impact and place minimal stress on joints. This makes them suitable for individuals with joint concerns or those recovering from injuries.

Isometric holds can be incorporated seamlessly into a busy schedule. Short, focused sessions can yield significant benefits, making it an excellent option for individuals with time constraints.

Isometric training encourages a strong mind-muscle connection. Focusing on engaging specific muscles during static holds enhances awareness and control over your body.

Before starting an isometric training program, it's essential to consider individual health factors. Consulting with a healthcare provider or fitness professional can ensure a safe and tailored approach.

Progressive overload is key to ongoing improvement. Gradually increasing the intensity, duration, or complexity of isometric exercises ensures continued challenge and growth.

Isometric training can seamlessly complement other forms of exercise, including dynamic strength training, cardiovascular workouts, and flexibility training. Combining these modalities enhances overall fitness.

Isometric training allows for a personalized approach based on fitness level, goals, and specific health considerations. Tailoring your routine ensures a program that aligns with your unique needs.

To experience the full benefits of isometric training, consistency is crucial. Regular practice, combined with proper rest and recovery, contributes to lasting results.

whether you're aiming to build foundational strength, improve joint stability, or enhance overall fitness, isometric training provides a valuable and adaptable tool. By incorporating these exercises thoughtfully into your routine and considering individual health factors, you can embark on a journey towards improved strength, stability, and a healthier lifestyle.

THE END